THE

GASTRIC SLEEVE

DIET GUIDE

------------------~----------------

A Comprehensive Gastric Sleeve Weight Loss Surgery Diet Guide

------------------~----------------

ALSO INCLUDES: KEYS, TIPS AND GOALS FOR SUCCESSFUL WEIGHT MAINTENANCE

BY

MONIKA SHAH

COPYRIGHT © 2016

A Message for Readers!

Heal Your New Stomach with the Right Diet & Care

This book has been specifically designed and written for people who are either planning for, or have already undergone the Gastric Sleeve surgery (Bariatric Surgery) for weight loss. This book will educate you in detail about the various stages of Gastric Sleeve surgery and help you sail through the healing period of weight loss surgery.

Let's take a closer look on what this book has to offer:

- **Part A – The Research**: This part of the book educates you not only about the Gastric Sleeve surgery itself but other various types of Bariatric surgeries too. It talks about the various risks and complications that are involved in this procedure. It also explains the various hospital procedures and processes one has to follow during the entire surgery along with the costs. Finally, it makes sure that you understand the right methods of selecting the best surgeon for your surgery too.

- **Part B – Getting Ready for the Surgery:** This part of the book prepares you for the Gastric Sleeve surgery by explaining the various guidelines that one has to follow before the surgery. It also talks about how you can maximize your success rate, various pre-operative diet guidelines including the 10 – 14 days Low Sugar diet. Finally, it helps you understand what you should take to the hospital along with you for those critical first few post-operative days.

- **Part C – The Maintenance and Care:** This is an important and critical part of the book which educates you in detail about the post-operative diet stages. You will explore the detailed post-surgery dietary information that one should follow to sail through the healing period of weight loss surgery. For each of these diet stages, book will unfold the real goals, guidelines, diet control measures and foods to eat and avoid from various food groups in detail.

It makes sure that the person who needs to be on Gastric Sleeve diet is well-versed with the required dietary information and guidelines to live a healthy and comfortable life.

Also Includes: Keys, Tips and Goals for Successful Weight Maintenance

When recovering after sleeve gastrectomy or any other form of bariatric surgery, patients also need to make some emotional adjustments. This section will help you with not only motivating yourself but also the keys, tips and goals one must follow for successful weight maintenance.

CONTENTS

Copyright Notes & Disclaimer

This Page Has Been Left Blank Intentionally.

PART A – THE RESEARCH

This Page Has Been Left Blank Intentionally.

Chapter 1

Understanding the Bariatric Surgery

How does it Work?

Often it becomes extremely difficult to treat severe obesity just with exercise and diet. In such situations doctors recommend bariatric surgery. It's a surgical procedure carried out on the stomach and/or intestines of extremely obese patients with the aim of helping them lose weight. Bariatric surgery is also often recommended when obese patients start suffering from serious health issues related to excess body weight.

This surgery works by restricting an individual's food intake and thereby results in weight loss. Patients undergoing the procedure also experience reduction in their chances of developing type-2 diabetes. There are also some types of bariatric surgery that work by interrupting the process of digestion and preventing nutrients like vitamin and a portion of the total calories consumed from getting absorbed.

Findings of recent studies are suggesting that bariatric surgery might even play a significant role in lowering death rates among severely obese patients. However, for this process to show best results patients must exercise regularly and adopt healthy dietary habits following the surgery.

Bariatric Surgery for Adults

At this moment, bariatric surgery is one of the most common ways of treating severely obese adults. Here, it must be mentioned that an individual's level of obesity is decided based on his or her BMI or body mass index, which is actually a measure of weight with respect to a person's height.

An adult is called severely obese if his/her BMI is 40 or more or if he/she has a serious obesity-related health problem along with a BMI of 35 or more. Examples of obesity-related health issues that might prompt doctors to recommend bariatric surgery include heart disease, acute sleep apnea (patients with sleep apnea experience one or more pauses in breathing while they sleep), type 2 diabetes etc.

Although it was not permitted previously, the FDA now allows doctors to use an AGB or adjustable gastric band for treating patients with a minimum of one obesity-related health disorder (for instance, diabetes or heart disease) and BMI of 30 or more.

Who Is An Ideal Adult Candidate?

Before undergoing surgery for producing weight loss, the candidate must be aware of every single step the process involves. Patients panning to undergo the operation should find answers to the following questions.

- Is it unlikely that he/she would lose weight or keep the excess weight off successfully for a long period of time using other techniques?

- Is he/she aware of all the effects of the surgery?

- Is he/she ready for losing weight and improving health?

- Does he/she know how the post-surgery life would be? (Patients undergoing this operation need to chew food well for enabling proper digestion and usually lose their ability of eating large meals.)

- Does the person know about the dietary restrictions the surgery will impose on him/her?

- Is the person ready to follow a strict diet plan, stay physically active (exercising regularly is a must), undergo medical follow-ups and consume additional minerals and vitamins for the rest of his/her life?

It must be noted that there's no method (this includes surgery) that can guarantee weight loss and prevention of a rebound. There are patients, who fail to achieve the desired weight loss, even after undergoing bariatric surgery. This can happen due to a number of reasons including problems such as separated stitches, a stretched pouch and so on. There are also many patients, who regain a portion of the weight they lost, over time. How much weight a patient would regain tends to vary depending on his/her level of obesity and the kind of surgery he/she underwent.

Bariatric Surgery for Youth

The recent years have seen significant increase in the rate of obesity among the country's youth. Young individuals suffering from extreme obesity are often treated with bariatric surgery. It's true that this surgery can help teens to lose weight, but there are still some questions about the long-term impact of the procedure on their developing minds and bodies.

Who Is An Ideal Youth Candidate?

According to bariatric surgery and childhood obesity experts, families should consider surgery only for teenagers, who have tried to lose weight using other methods (for instance, diet and exercise) for at least six months, but haven't had any success. Some other criteria the candidates should meet include:

- They should be extremely obese (must have a BMI of 40 or more).

- The candidate must be at his/her adult height (for girls it usually happens when they are 13 or older and for boys the age is typically 15 or older).

- The candidate must be suffering from serious obesity-related health problems, for instance, sleep apnea and type-2 diabetes.

Other than considering the above factors, healthcare providers must also assess how prepared the teens and their parents are for the operation and the lifestyle changes to be incorporated following the process. For best results, these young patients must undergo the surgery at bariatric surgery centers meant for the youth. These centers are run with the aim of meeting special requirements of young people.

Evidence collected from clinical studies conducted over the years suggests that weight loss surgery can help teens suffering from extreme obesity both in losing weight and becoming healthier. Statistics also reveal that gastric bypass surgery is the most commonly used operation for treating severe obesity in the youth. The eight years between 1996 and 2003 have witnessed around 2,700 youth undergo bariatric surgeries.

Experts suggest that this procedure is as safe for the teens as it is for the adults. Here, it must be noted that the US FDA still doesn't allow use of AGB for individuals below the age of 18 years. However, AGB has been found to offer positive weight-loss results when used to treat obese youth in foreign lands.

Types & Risks of Weight Loss Surgeries

There are a variety of weight loss surgeries that can be performed on individuals. Each weight loss surgery comes with its own benefits and risks which makes it important for people to know about not only the benefits but the associated risks. Let's now understand these various weight loss surgeries and their associated risks one by one.

Sleeve Gastrectomy

In this kind of restrictive surgery, the Bariatric surgeon will separate a small section of your stomach and remove it from your body. The portion left behind is given the approximate shape of a tube. Apart from the fact that your 'revised' stomach will not be able to contain much food, the surgery will also, reduce the production of ghrelin (appetite-regulating hormone).

Sleeve Gastrectomy is a relatively new procedure in comparison to the others. Here are some of the risks associated with this type of surgery.

- It is possible that the sleeve (tube) become dilated over the years, preventing sufficient weight loss.

- However, the biggest risk associated with this procedure is leakage. If this happens, you might require a second surgery, along with the placement of a feeding tube and a drainage tube. The tubes are temporary.

- Persistent leaks may lead to the formation of wounds or abscesses, thereby prompting a lengthy stay at the hospital.

- Wounds and infections may be treated with powerful antibiotics, but there is always the possibility of further complications.

- Then again, if you are prone towards heavy bleeding after the operation, you may require a blood transfusion.

- A careless surgeon may cause damage to the organs close to the operation site. If this should happen, you will require additional operative procedures.

- Although rare, it is possible that your 'revised' gut is unable to tolerate sufficient amounts of food. You will have to go in for total parenteral nutrition (TPN) then, that is, fed via intravenous methods.

- You may find a few blood clots accumulating in legs and traveling to your lungs. It happens rarely, but can prove fatal.

- Stay away from this procedure if you suffer from frequent heartburn.

Laparoscopic Adjustable Gastric Banding

This restrictive procedure involves fixing a band with an inflatable balloon around the upper region of your stomach. The balloon is akin to a pouch with a narrow opening, which leads to the lower portion of your stomach. Next, the surgeon will place a port possessing a tube, under the skin of your abdomen. The tube acts as the connection between the band and the port. You will be able to deflate or inflate the balloon by removing or injecting fluid through this port. Thus, your gastric band may be adjusted according to will.

Laparoscopic Adjustable Gastric Banding offers the following risks.

- You need not worry too much if you should experience diarrhea, constipation, regurgitation, acid reflux, or nausea, after the operation. You will be all right soon. Rush to the Emergency Room only if abdominal pain persists for a long time, such as beyond three hours.

- Leakage is an issue with this kind of surgery too; your Band may begin to leak. You may require a repeat operation.

- It is possible for the new implant to migrate and cause complications. This refers to displacement of the port, band erosion, or the band slipping from its place.

- Sometimes, the port becomes detached from the tubing, leading to all kinds of complications.

- Of course, like with any other surgical procedure, the site of the operation may become infected. Similarly, your stomach or esophagus may experience inflammation too. Antibiotics should help.

- It is quite possible for your esophagus to go into a spasm after the operation. However, this is not commonly witnessed.

- If you suffer from gastro-esophageal reflux disease (GERD), please avoid this type of surgery.

Duodenal Switch with Biliopancreatic Diversion

This malabsorptive surgery begins with the removal of a large portion of your stomach. What is left behind is the stomach valve responsible for sending food to the small intestine, as well as the duodenum (first part of small intestine). The Bariatric surgeon will close off the middle part of your small intestine. Thus, it becomes possible to connect the duodenum and the last part of the small intestine directly, thereby creating the duodenal switch. The Biliopancreatic diversion is created by re-connecting the separated middle section to the last section of the small intestine. This permits pancreatic and bile juices to flow into this region.

Duodenal Switch with Biliopancreatic Diversion also carries the same risks of infection along the staple line, leakage into the abdomen, and formation of blood clots in the legs and lungs. Apart from these, there are some specific long-term and short-term risks too.

- You might suffer from something known as the Dumping Syndrome, caused by an inability to tolerate processed sugars or highly refined and high-calorie foodstuffs. As soon as you consume sweet-tasting stuff, you experience nausea, cramping, sweating, extreme fatigue, dizziness or lightheadedness and heart palpitations. Explosive diarrhea can weaken you to such an extent that you have to lie down for some time.

- It is also possible to become a victim of frequent diarrhea and foul smelling stools, because your gut finds it difficult to absorb vitamins, protein, fats, iron and calcium.

- It follows that you will experience nutritional deficiency, as you become habituated to eating lesser and lesser food. You may have to consume vitamin supplements throughout your life.

- When you are nutritionally deficient, your bones become weak. Thus, you are at high risk for osteoporosis.

Roux-en-Y Gastric Bypass

This malabsorptive surgery comprises of the creation of a small pouch on the top of your stomach. All the food that you consume will enter this pouch only, and go nowhere else. However, digestive juices will continue to be made in your main stomach region. The surgeon will ensure that the portions of the small intestine present below the main stomach and attached to it, respectively, are cut and attached to the new pouch, as well as to one another.

Roux-en-Y Gastric Bypass tends to cause death in one amongst 200 patients (0.5% risk). Therefore, you should discuss this elective procedure thoroughly with your Bariatric surgeon before you proceed with it.

- Apart from the possibility of infection at the site of surgery, formation of blood clots, vitamin deficiency or leakage into the abdominal cavity, you may even become anemic or develop osteoporosis.

- Sometimes, your gallbladder is also removed during the surgical process. In case, it is not, gallstones may accumulate within it. The doctor will advise the consumption of preventive medications.

- If you do not drink sufficient water, you might get kidney stones.

- It is possible for your intestine to twist around itself, thereby causing hernia.

- You may require a second operation to resolve issues related to the newly created pouch or strictures (connections become too narrow).

- Frequent failure to adhere to changes in diet or lifestyle, may lead to weight gain instead of weight loss.

Do not be under the impression that a surgical process is the ultimate cure for something chronic. Even a tried-and-proven method may be associated with some complications. The intention is not to frighten you. You are merely being advised to acquire clarity about any operation that you wish to undergo.

This Page Has Been Left Blank Intentionally.

Chapter 2

The Gastric Sleeve Complications

Complications from sleeve gastrectomy are pretty rare, but are usually much more serious compared to other weight loss procedures like gastric banding. For instance, occurrence of a leak during the process might turn out to be a serious problem that can take weeks or even months to subside.

Gastric sleeve surgery is a fairly new weight loss method. So, at this moment, it is very difficult to gather enough log-term data (facts and figures obtained for a period of more than 10 years) that would help us to understand what would happen with the weight loss. Many experts believe that with time, the sleeve will start dilating and the weight loss will no more be as impressive as it used to be after a couple of years following the surgery.

Like any other major surgery, sleeve gastrectomy also comes with a risk profile. Patients planning to undergo the process as well as their respective families must comprehend the profile before proceeding. The list bellow includes all the issues a patient can face after undergoing this weight loss surgery. This extensive list has not been prepared with the aim of worrying you. It will just provide you with a clear idea about different complications the method is linked to irrespective of how rare they are.

Acute Complications

- **Leaks on staple line:** Around one in every 100 patients undergoing the procedure experiences this complication. At times, the patients might need to get a repeat surgery done for allowing the problem to subside. The repeat operation is usually carried out within the first few days following the original procedure. Doctors might extend the length of the patient's hospital stay if he or she is found to be suffering from this issue (the stay might be extended by weeks and if required by months). If left untreated, these leaks might lead to serious conditions such as abscesses and fistula.

- **Bleeding:** Patients might suffer from postoperative bleeding and may need blood transfusion to get rid of the problem. This issue is also often managed by reoperation. Around 1 in 200 patients experience bleeding after sleeve gastrectomy.

- **Infection:** Infections following the surgery are managed occasionally with reoperation and mostly with antibiotics.

- **Organ damage:** Like any other keyhole process, this one can also see the patient suffer an accidental injury to organs close to the operated region. Your doctor might recommend a repeat surgery for repairing the injured organs.

- **Wound issues:** Obese individuals or people with high BMI tend to remain at extremely high risk of developing wound infections and haematomas. High BMI also result in impaired wound healing in these patients.

- **Blood clots:** Sleeve gastrectomy can be followed by conditions such as pulmonary embolus (marked by blood clotting in lungs) and deep venous thromboses (marked by blood clotting in veins).

- **Chest infections or pneumonia**

- **Other rare issues:** Gastric sleeve surgery works by changing the function of our gut. This change in function often ends up impairing the patient's ability of tolerating adequate food intakes. Individuals who face this problem are treated with TPN or total parenteral nutrition, a process involving continuous supply of nutrition by means of intravenous methods.

Long Term Complications

- Like all other intra-abdominal methods involving the patient's gastrointestinal tract, this one can also be linked with long term health issues related to adhesions or scar tissue in the gut. To get rid of the problem, the patient might need to undergo another operation.

- Like other intra-abdominal methods, sleeve gastrectomy also leaves the patient at mild risk of developing hernia. Repeat surgery is the most commonly used solution to this problem.

- The patient's chances of having heartburn or gastro-esophageal reflux disease (GERD) may increase. Postoperative reflux is often treated with acid suppressing medications. Around one in five patients experience symptoms of GERD after one year of undergoing the operation. On the other hand, around 3% of patients experience the symptoms after three years of the surgery.

  Doctors usually don't recommend gastric sleeve surgery to patients with history of reflux.

- Occasionally, the surgery might also cause malabsorption of different micronutrient. The problem can be managed easily with supplemental minerals and vitamins. In addition, the patient must be monitored through regular blood tests.

Data collected in the past few years suggest that although very rarely, death from sleeve gastrectomy is also possible. However, at 0.19%, the mortality rate is pretty low.

It has been found that in most cases, patients are responsible for developing postoperative complications. Thus, if you are planning to undergo sleeve gastrectomy, the first thing you must do is educating yourself and the members of your family about the procedure.

Chapter 3

The Costs & General Hospital Procedures

The Costs

Your location is the primary deciding factor when it comes to the amount of money you will have to spend for undergoing gastric sleeve surgery. The cost of this particular type of bariatric surgery is actually slightly less than gastric bypass surgery and slightly more than gastric band surgery. The year 2015 saw an overall drop of 5% in the price of this weight loss surgery compared to what it was in 2014. However, during this period, the drop has been more prominent in the 10 most expensive US states. Those states have experienced a drop of 10% on average. This reduction in price has taken place possibly due to the growing demand of the procedure.

- The pricing ranges between $9,600 and $26,000 across the United States

- The most frequently quoted price for the process is $14,900

- The average (rounded up) price of the surgery in the country is $16,800.

Here, it must be noted that all the prices mentioned above are 'cash pay' prices i.e. prices to be paid by people who are not using insurance for covering the cost of the surgery. These people either make payments in cash or by using their debit or credit card. It might surprise you, but the fact is that the cash price for sleeve gastrectomy is less than the amount the hospital would make the insurance company pay.

Here, it must be noted that sleeve gastrectomy was originally not a medical procedure covered by insurance. Insurance companies used to pay for the surgery only if the doctors had to carry it out as part of another procedure called staged gastric bypass. However, now after witnessing great successes achieved by sleeve gastrectomy, many top insurance companies have started offering cover for this surgery as a primary weight loss procedure.

One question that may come to your mind when preparing for gastric sleeve surgery is that does lower price always mean that you are being benefited. Getting the operation done for a lower price is definitely good news, but that's not the only factor that decides whether or not you are getting the best treatment. Some factors that will play major role in this journey of yours are who will be performing the operation, where it will be performed, how much money you are willing to spend etc. Cost is actually just one factor. It is definitely not the sole factor.

Does a low price indicate that the surgeon is less qualified or skilled? It's true that it would not be wise to sacrifice a surgeon's skill and experience over price when undergoing a major surgical procedure like sleeve gastrectomy. However, it must also be mentioned that low price doesn't indicate that the surgeon operating you is less qualified or less skilled compared to the surgeons who charge bigger amounts. Often, the cost of surgeries is decided by hospitals and has nothing to do with the surgeon's expertise. There are also many surgeons who want to help patients by offering their lowest possible prices. There are also surgeons, who keep their charges low to bring in more patients.

Hospital Procedures for Bariatric Surgeries

You cannot just walk into a Bariatric clinic and admit yourself as a patient. You will have to submit to an in-depth evaluation conducted by experienced professionals first. They are part of a multidisciplinary team, which takes into account your existing physical condition, mental status, nutritional habits and lifestyle, before selecting or rejecting you for surgery.

Some institutes set up general seminars, in order to disseminate information about Bariatric surgery. Such informative sessions help you to prepare yourself better for what might lie ahead, as well as, create a list of questions that you might like answered by the surgeon concerned.

Regardless of whether you attend such a seminar or not, you will have to take the help of your primary care provider for setting up an appointment with a Bariatric surgeon. After the appointment is fixed, you may have to fill up certain documents with details about your personal history, past medical history, current medications, allergies, etc. You will have to submit them to the Bariatric surgeon during the initial consultation.

After going through these forms during the first consultation, the Bariatric surgeon may request further information about your existing co-morbidities. Do not leave out any details of your past or present experiences. Rest assured; there will be no breach of confidentiality. You would not like to invite further complications in your life by leaving out vital information, would you?

Once the assessment is complete and the surgeon has clarified all your doubts, he/she will provide information about the kind of surgery procedure that is most suitable for you. Yes, even the risks associated with it will be discussed. Finally, you will be requested to undergo certain tests, such as complete blood picture, electrocardiogram to discover the condition of your heart, screening for diabetes, etc. In case, you suffer from sleep apnea, you will have to undergo a sleep study.

Mere physical and laboratory evaluations will not suffice to categorize you as a suitable patient for bariatric surgery. You will need to undergo a psychological assessment too. It is imperative that the psychologist comprehend how your choices and quality of life have been affected by your "weighty" problems. After all, you have to be willing to make major changes in your life after the surgery. You cannot afford to be emotionally weak. In fact, the counselor may even advise you to take certain medications to improve your mental status, as well as make appointments for regular psychotherapy sessions, if the situation warrants it.

Does the dietitian have a role to play in this scenario? Yes, he/she definitely has! In fact, you will have to set up several sessions with this well-qualified and well-trained expert, prior to your surgery. Provide her with every single detail about your past dietary habits and your attempts at losing excess weight. Armed with this information, he/she will be able to provide guidance regarding the new eating habits that have to be adopted after Bariatric surgery. If you are serious about weight loss, you will need to have tips about the diet regimen to be followed at home, what foodstuffs to choose when you eat out, how your choices influence your stress levels and moods, etc.

When the results of all your tests and evaluations have been submitted to the Bariatric surgeon, he/she will invite you for a final consult. The details of the surgery under question and the complications associated with it will also be discussed once again. If everything proves satisfactory, the doctor will request your approval for the surgery. Do not worry; you will be granted some time to think everything over and get back at your convenience.

Every hospital has its rules and regulations, as well as its unique payment structure. Some of the staff may be deemed as visiting staff; they demand their own fees. Therefore, whether you do so during the initial consult or final meeting, do not forget to request details about the costs associated with the surgery, hospital stay, post-operative care, etc. Note that you are going in for elective (not compulsory) surgery, not something that is imperative to improve your health.

Your insurance company may not be willing to finance you 100%; you will have to share the expenses. Take the assistance of the administrative staff at the concerned clinic for dealing with your insurance coverage, as well as requesting pre-authorization for your surgical procedure. They will even supply supporting documents with your insurance forms, to strengthen your case. On your part, you have to be patient. Some insurance companies provide approval rapidly, while others take over a month to do so.

When everything has been resolved to satisfaction, you may fix a date for your surgery. A week before that, you will have to submit to a thorough physical examination and pre-admission testing.

This Page Has Been Left Blank Intentionally.

Chapter 4

The Surgeon Selection

If you want the surgery to show best possible results, you must get it done by an experienced and reputable surgeon. The tips below will help you find the best gastric sleeve surgeon in your area.

- If you are getting ready to undergo sleeve gastrectomy, you should opt for a bariatric surgeon, who specializes in this particular type of weight loss surgery. He/she should have a minimum of ten years of experience of carrying out such operations and must have an impressive success rate. Studies have shown that if the surgeon conducting these operations has several years of experience behind him/her, the patient's chances of developing complications after the procedure drops significantly.

  If you get the surgery done by a team of surgeons associated with a reputable hospital in your area, your chances of getting the desired results will be significantly high.

- If you are in America, the surgeon you choose must be certified either by the American Osteopathic Board of Surgery or by the American Board of Surgery. These board certifications indicate that the surgeon succeeded in meeting some specific standards and completed a related training program. These certifications need to be renewed once in every ten years.

- Your bariatric surgeon must be certified by the ASMBS (American Society for Metabolic & Bariatric Surgery) and must have performed at least 25 surgeries as the main surgeon during the past couple of years.

- Don't forget to ask the surgeon whether he/she will be accompanied by another doctor during the operation. If the answer is yes, you must also check the credentials (experience, qualification etc.) of the assistant.

It's also extremely important to get the surgery done at a trustworthy hospital or nursing home. The place must be known for offering the best possible care to overweight and obese patients. The care required by these people is usually much different from that of patients with normal body weight.

The facility picked by you must have the experience of meeting the special needs of obese and overweight individuals. It must have the right set of equipment, for instance, bigger blood pressure cuffs, sufficiently sized CT scanners, wider hospital beds, larger operating tables and wheelchair toilets, and extra-large (or even bigger) gowns.

Anesthesia is known to cause some specific complications in obese patients. So, the facility must also have anesthesiologists, who have the experience of dealing with obese individuals.

Before getting yourself admitted to the hospital, you must also check the kind of support they will offer you after the surgery. As you will read the book, you will know that the surgery is actually the beginning of your weight loss journey. How much success it will bring for you, depends primarily on aftercare. It would be of great help if the hospital you are getting operated at offers services like psychological counseling, support groups, physical therapy or exercise, nutrition counseling etc.

This Page Has Been Left Blank Intentionally.

PART B –GETTING READY FOR THE SURGERY

This Page Has Been Left Blank Intentionally.

Chapter 5

Preparing for the Gastric Sleeve Surgery

This chapter will help you to prepare yourself for the surgery. Here, you will get to know about the items you should take to the hospital, things you shouldn't do before the surgery and foods you must consume when getting yourself ready for the method.

Maximizing Your Success Rate

The preparation for this surgical procedure includes a number of steps. These steps help in optimizing the patient's body for undergoing the operation.

The patient must be extremely careful about personal hygiene. This is essential for reducing the chances of postoperative infection. He or she should not skip daily baths (using a high quality soap is a must during this phase) for at least a month before the surgery. When bathing, the person must be extra attentive when cleaning the abdominal region (from the breasts to the groin). Special care is also needed when cleaning the skin folds.

Maintaining good oral hygiene is also extremely important. The patient must brush and floss his/her teeth twice every day on a regular basis

It is mandatory that the patient starts following a strict diet plan when preparing for the process. Including exercise into daily routine would also be helpful. Doctors say that even minor weight loss prior to the operation might make the stomach's surgical exposure safer and easier. Another benefit of altering eating habits and getting started with an exercise program before the operation is that the patient will find it easier to cope with the changes introduced during the postoperative phase.

Different surgeons recommend different kinds of preoperative diet. So, you will most likely receive detailed instructions about the diet plan you will have to follow from your surgeon's office. They will also tell you from when you should start following that diet.

Two Weeks Prior the Surgery

- Don't take arthritis medications, ibuprofen and aspirin for at least a couple of weeks prior to the surgery. This is because these medications increase an individual's chances of bleeding.

- If you are on birth control pills or taking estrogen hormones in any other form, you should inform your surgeon about that.

- Stop taking all OTC and prescription appetite suppressants a couple of weeks before the operation.

Individuals, who are not sure which medications should be stopped, should consult the surgeon. Is your life still inactive? If yes, then this is the best time to add some kind of activity in it. You can start going for a walk every morning or evening or join a swimming class. Just five to 10 minutes of activity per day before the surgery will help you immensely.

When you are just a couple of weeks away from the day of surgery, having the following items at home may help. Some of these items will come in handy even after the surgery.

- A food processor or blender
- Mineral and vitamin supplements (consult the surgeon's office before buying)
- Broth
- Non-carbonated, caffeine-free, calorie-free beverages
- Powdered, sugar-free diet beverage mix
- Seasonings and flavorings like True Orange, True Lemon, True Lime
- Non-carbonated, sugar free, zero calorie spring water
- Calorie-free sugar substitute
- Decaffeinated tea or coffee
- Protein supplements

Two Days before the Surgery

Two days prior to the surgery, you must stop eating or drinking anything after midnight. You must even stay away from cigarettes, breath mints and gum. Keep clear liquids ready. You will need them during the stage 1 of the postoperative phase. These liquid protein supplements can be easily obtained from both online shops and local stores. Go for low carbohydrate, high protein whey protein powder (buy the unflavored powder). Other items you can try include strawberry sorbet, chicken soup, lemonade etc. You must consume protein powders by adding them to a clear liquid beverage or water.

Pre-Op 10-14 Days Low Sugar Diet

Your surgeon might ask you to follow a liquid, low-sugar diet for 10 to 14 days before the surgery. Such recommendations are made for depleting the glycogen stored in patients' liver and making the laparoscopic surgery simpler. Preoperative low sugar diet is also known to alleviate the risk of serious complications.

Another benefit of following this diet is that it helps in shrinking fat depositions around different organs, which can make you a more suitable candidate for sleeve gastrectomy or any other laparoscopy surgery.

If your surgeon has asked you to follow a liquid, low sugar diet for 10 to 14 days prior to the operation, you will find the following guidelines helpful.

1. You should consume the liquids mentioned below in moderation (max 2 cups a day) as their sugar content is high:

   - PowerAde
   - G2 Gatorade
   - Juice (opt for juices with low sugar content, for instance, tomato juice, grapefruit juice, orange juice or apple juice)

2. The following liquids should be limited to 3 or less servings a day:

- Popsicles
- Regular Jell-o
- Zero sugar Fudgesicles

3. Have 3 or less servings of the following every day:

  - 6 ounces fat-free/light yogurt
  - 1 cup milk (Lactaid, skim or soy)
  - ½ cup cottage cheese (low fat)

4. Take 2 to 3 servings of any high quality protein shake (ask your surgeon to recommend).

5. You can take any amount of the following liquids as they don't contain sugar:

  - Tea or coffee with zero calorie sugar substitute
  - Sugar-free, noncarbonated beverages
  - Vegetable/beef/chicken broth
  - Sugar-free Jell-O and popsicles

Here, it must be noted that during the postoperative liquid stages, you will not be allowed to consume Fudgesicles and other beverages containing sugar in any amount. During those stages, your surgeon will only allow you to have zero calorie beverages and protein supplements.

A Sample Menu for the Liquid, Low Sugar Pre-Op Diet

Breakfast

- Orange juice- 1 cup
- Coffee (you can add 2 teaspoons non-dairy powdered creamer and zero calorie sugar substitute)- 1 cup

Mid-Morning

- Protein shake (combine 6 to 8 oz. water, ½ cup low soy or skim milk, 1 scoop protein powder and ice and blend it in a shaker cup or blender)

Lunch

- Beef or chicken broth- 1 cup
- Jell-O gelatin- 6 oz. (opt for the regular variety, you can use fat-free yogurt as topping)
- Gatorade G2 (low sugar)- 1 cup

Mid-Afternoon

- Protein shake (prepare it in the same manner as described above)
- Sugar-free Popsicle or Jell-O

Dinner

- Fat free/light yogurt- 6 oz or
- Cottage cheese (low fat)- ½ cup
- Protein shake (prepare it in the same manner as described above)
- Orange Sunrise
- Jell-O gelatin- 6 oz (the regular variety)

Bedtime

- Zero sugar Fudgesicle- 1
- If you want you can have a serving of protein shake (this time prepare it just by blending 1 scoop protein powder and 8 to 16 oz of water) or a sugar-free drink with ice

In between the main meals of the day you can have all the sugar-free liquids mentioned above.

What to Bring To the Hospital and What Not?

The majority of the top hospitals will not need you to bring anything with you. However, if you want you can bring the following items with you.

- A pillow
- Slippers and robe

- A couple of underwear (you will need them during the 2nd and 3rd day after the surgery)
- Shampoo (your surgeon will allow you to shower 2 or 3 days after the surgery)
- Clothes (you will need them when leaving the hospital)
- Lip balm or chap stick
- If you are a menstruating female, carry feminine hygiene products (you may get your cycle before time due to stress caused by the surgery)
- Bipap or C-pap machines

Don't bring any of the medications you take at home with you. You will not need them at the hospital.

PART C- THE MAINTENANCE AND CARE

This Page Has Been Left Blank Intentionally.

Chapter 6

Post Surgery: The First Few Days

Following the surgery patients are shifted to the PACU or Post Anesthesia Recovery Area. Their oxygen saturation, blood pressure and heart rate are monitored constantly. To ensure that the patients don't suffer from severe pain (it's impossible to make patients absolutely pain free, but the intensity of pain can be made tolerable) even after the effects of anesthesia subside, a pain medication is directly injected into the patients' intravenous (IV) line.

At times, patients are also allowed to use PCA pumps or patient-controlled pain medication buttons. However, for that they will have to be fully conscious.

A nurse will teach you the process of using PCA pumps. Pain medications administered by PCA buttons are known to show quick results, typically within minutes. The PCA pumps come equipped with timers, which will ensure that you are receiving your doses accurately. They will never allow you to become a victim of overdose. Overdose of pain killers are known to cause a series of debilitating side effects. Here, it must be noted that you may feel sleepy after receiving the medicine. The PCA pump cannot be operated by the patients' visitors, which even include their family members.

If required, you will be given oxygen by means of nasal prongs or mask. The nurse will make you wear air stockings, which will deflate and inflate alternatively for preventing blood clots. You should not remove these stocking even when walking.

After spending a few hours at the PACU, you will be shifted to a regular room in the hospital. If a patient develops serious complications after the surgery, he or she might be shifted to the ICU (intensive care unit).

After getting adjusted to the new room, you will be asked to practice breathing exercises (10 times each hour when awake). You will have to perform the exercises using incentive spirometer. Ideally, a family member should be with you overnight.

Place a pillow in a way so that it splints your abdomen perfectly and keep coughing and breathing deeply. Coughing might make you feel a bit uncomfortable, but will never injure the surgical site. If there's no complication, you will be allowed to get up and walk in the same evening, but with assistance from your nurse.

Day 1 after Surgery

You should continue coughing and breathing deeply using your pillow as the tool for splinting your abdomen. The nurse will encourage you to walk around your room. Doing this will help you in preventing formation of blood clots and averting conditions like pneumonia. On the 1st day following the surgery, your nurse will be assisting you to get up from the bed and walk in the room several times. She will also assist you to regulate pain medication.

On the same day, you will be receiving injections of a medicine meant for preventing blood clots. These injections will be given in your abdomen using extremely small needles. If you are a patient without any serious health complication, you can expect your urinary catheter to be removed on the 1st postoperative day.

You may need to undergo a swallow test. It's a diagnostic test that will need you to swallow a dye to allow doctors confirm that there's no leak in your abdomen. If the healthcare providers are happy with the results of your swallow test, you will be served with ice chips and clear liquids.

Some patients don't need to undergo the swallow test. However, they will also be kept on a liquid diet. On the first day following the surgery, they will get to eat water, broth, crystal light and Jell-O (sugar free).

Patients should avoid eating fast. They should take at least 30 to 40 minutes to finish the liquids. It's not mandatory to consume everything you are served with. Only have as much as you can. Remember that the majority of the patients undergoing this surgery can't eat properly for several days and at times for several weeks following the operation.

Day 2 after Surgery

If there's no complication, you should be able to walk around the hall on the 2nd day after the operation. You should visit the hall for walking four times during that day. Walking plays an extremely important role in preventing postoperative complications like blood clotting and pneumonia.

Sip water at regular intervals. You should consume only as much as you can without stressing yourself. Your nurse will definitely keep the water pitcher in your room filled so that you can continue sipping all through the day. If you take medications for other health problems, you will also have to start taking them, but either in liquid or in crushed form.

Surgeons typically allow patients undergoing sleeve gastrectomy to take shower from the 2nd day following the operation. If you are allowed to do so, don't forget to cover your incisions using a plastic wrap before getting into the shower.

Your discharge teaching will also begin on the 2nd postoperative day. A dietician might visit you and share his/her suggestions with you.

Day 3 after Surgery

Some patients are discharged on day 2. However, if you were not discharged on the 2nd postoperative day, you will surely get discharged on day 3 (unless there's any serious complication)

Before being discharged, you will receive a series of instructions from healthcare providers at the hospital. They will explain your home care routine in detail. You will get ample opportunity to clear all your confusions. You may be asked to take prescription pain medications and antiulcer medications at home.

Patients, who are suffering from a fever or are struggling to consume enough liquid or a have been diagnosed with any health complication, might need to stay one or two extra days at the hospital.

Don't forget to get yourself checked by the surgeon 7 to 10 days following the surgery.

Never ignore health complications such as leg or chest pain and acute breathing problem. This is because they might be indicators of blood clotting. If you experience any of those signs after returning home, call your surgeon right away. You can also visit a nearby emergency room to get yourself checked. A fever of more than 101 must also be reported promptly at the surgeon's office.

This Page Has Been Left Blank Intentionally.

Chapter 7

Post Surgery: Diet Advancements

Stage 1 to Stage 4

The Four Stages

Once your gastric sleeve surgery is done, you will have to go through four stages of diet. Usually, the surgeon or a dietician recommended by him/her provides the patients detailed information about the changes they will have to make in their diet in each of these four stages.

Stage 1: In this stage, patients are only allowed to drink clear liquids. Stage 1 starts at the hospital and persists for a couple of weeks. Patients in this stage get nutrition from clear liquid protein supplements.

Stage 2: In stage 2, patients are required to be on a full liquid diet. Like stage 1, this stage also lasts for a couple of weeks. During these two weeks, your surgeon will allow you to have protein shakes along with the clear liquids you were having in stage 1.

Stage 3: Stage 3 is the stage of blended diet. It starts right after stage 2 and persists for two weeks.

Stage 4: Usually, stage 4 starts in week 7 and lasts until the patient succeeds in losing 75% of his/her excess body weight. When a patient achieves that goal, the dietician might add a few food items to his/her stage-4 diet. You should never add any extra food to your diet without consulting your surgeon or dietician. In fact, your surgeon or dietician will tell you how, when and what food items should be added. Here, it must be noted that the concepts adopted in stage 4 must be practiced by the patients for the rest of their lives.

Patients need to learn and practice healthy lifestyle behavior and dietary habits all through the first 12 months following the surgery. This process of learning should actually continue throughout their lifetime.

To ensure that you are on the right track, you must visit a certified dietician at regular intervals. Start with a meeting a few weeks prior to the surgery. The post-surgery follow up visits should occur after one week, six months, one year, 18 months and then once every year (or as advised by your surgeon). However, you should visit the surgeon's office more frequently for follow up.

After the surgery, your caffeine intake must be limited to 8 ounce or 1 to 2 cups of coffee a day. Here, it must be noted that caffeinated beverages don't replenish our body fluids.

You should drink carbonated beverages only with your surgeon's approval. Usually, surgeons introduce carbonated beverages around 6 months after the operation.

Protein Intake during the Postoperative Phase

Protein is the most vital nutrient for any individual who has undergone gastric sleeve. The pointers below would explain the reasons behind protein's importance.

- Protein promotes hair growth and wound healing. It also prevents hair loss.

- If you don't consume adequate protein after the surgery, your body will start burning muscle tissues instead of the stored fat.

- Protein aids maintenance of lean muscles.

- Consuming the right amount of protein is important to prevent fatigue.

Patients undergoing sleeve gastrectomy must consume 60 to 80 grams of protein every day. One ounce protein is equivalent to 7 grams of protein. For meeting the minimum daily requirement of 60 grams, you must consume 3 ounces of the nutrient at every meal (breakfast, lunch and dinner).

Even when in stage 1 and 2, you will need to consume protein in form of clear liquids (in stage 1) and protein shakes (in stage 2) for proper healing and nutrition.

Stage 1: Have Clear Liquids or Fluids

When in this stage, you should abide by the following guidelines:

- Avoid gulping the liquids, sip them slowly. If required, you can use a straw.

- Stay away from fruit juices as they contain lots of carbohydrates and calories. If you add fruit juice to your diet, your weight loss process will slow down.

- You can drink all noncarbonated, calorie free, sugar free and caffeine free beverages. They will help in replenishing your body fluids. Don't forget to read the nutrition labels of the products carefully. (If every 8 ounce serving of a beverage contains 0 to 5 calories, the beverage is categorized as calorie-free.)

You will need fluids consumed in stage 1 in every stage. Your surgeon will ask you to drink at least 64 ounces of fluid each day. However, that's just the minimum you must consume, it shouldn't be your goal. If you can drink more clear liquid, it would be good for your health.

Here are some fluids that can be used towards hydration:

- Vegetable, beef or chicken broth
- Decaf tea
- Decaf coffee
- Mio or Crystal Light

- Sugar free popsicles
- Water

Your dietician or surgeon might tell you names of some approved protein supplements that you can consume in stage 1. It has been found that during the first week after the surgery, patients tend to tolerate Nectar and Unjury best.

As mentioned above, stage 1 lasts for a couple of weeks, but you shouldn't move to the next stage without consulting your surgeon. It would be wise to purchase clear liquid protein supplements in bulk. The items should last for 10 to 14 days.

Stage 2- Stage of Full Liquids

Begin this stage only after your dietician or surgeon asks you to do so. Usually, it starts two weeks after the operation and lasts for another two weeks. In stage 2, you should stop consuming all clear liquid protein supplements that you were having in stage 1, unless your dietician or surgeon recommends otherwise. You should, however, continue drinking a minimum of 64 ounces of approved beverages. You can continue to have the same beverages you were having in stage 1. This is important as many full liquid protein supplements are not capable of replenishing your body fluids.

The full liquid protein supplements you will be having in stage 2 are the only beverages and food you will be allowed to take in this stage. Your healthcare providers will not allow you to consume anything else. However, they will ensure that you get your daily requirement of protein and calories from those supplements. You should never rush when drinking these supplements. Sip and gulp them slowly to avoid indigestion.

You might be asked to have these protein supplements even beyond stage 2 if your healthcare provider finds that you are constantly struggling to consume enough protein to meet your body's nutritional needs. In those advanced stages, your dietician might even ask you to replace any one major meal of the day with protein supplement. Here, it must be mentioned that you should not continue having these supplements in stage 3, stage 4 and beyond without asking your dietician or surgeon.

You will come across multiple brands of these protein supplements on the market. Follow the guidelines below before choosing a product for yourself. Asking your surgeon for a recommendation would also be wise.

- Search for a supplement that contains whey protein isolate. Our body absorbs this component more easily than whey protein concentrate (it contains milk sugar or lactose).

- Ideally, a serving of the supplement purchased by you should offer 20 grams protein.

- The product you pick should have less than 5g carbohydrate per serving.

- Supplements used in this stage might have milk-like consistency. You may get them in flavors like chocolate or vanilla. (However, you cannot have milk in stage 2. Milk, due to its carbohydrate content, might affect the weight loss process.)

- These supplements are either available as ready-to-drink solutions or as powders. It's up to you which type you would like to have.

Stage 3: Stage of Blended Diet

After following the full liquid diet plan of stage 2, ask your surgeon whether you can switch to stage 3. Move forward only if your surgeon asks you to do so. Like the previous two stages, this stage also persists for a couple of weeks.

When in this stage, you will need a blender or a food processor for preparing your meals. All the hard food items will have to be blended mechanically for giving them a finely chopped, smooth consistency. You will not need to blend the soft foods.

In stage 3, you will not be allowed to engage in snacking and will have to eat three meals every day. Your diet might not include the protein supplement you had in stage 2 unless you are facing troubles in meeting your protein needs consistently. If required, your surgeon might also use those supplements as meal replacements.

Stage 3 will need you to keep records of your daily food intake.

Another rule to be followed in stage 3 is that you will have to separate drinking and eating by at least 30 minutes. You should not consume any liquid 30 minutes prior to a meal. Similarly, after having your meal, you will have to wait for a minimum of 30 minutes before drinking liquids.

You should not try to eat quickly even in this stage. Ideally, you must take around 30 minutes to finish your meal.

If you want to exceed or meet your hydration goal of consuming at least 64 ounces of fluid every day, you must start sipping fluid very early in the morning. Continue sipping all through the day and you will surely not have any problem in exceeding the goal set by your surgeon.

In stage 3, each meal should contain a minimum of 20 grams or 3 ounces protein.

You should begin every meal with protein. Follow it up with low carb vegetables if you are still hungry after consuming your proteins. The vegetables are just meant for adding some variation to your meals. Having them is not mandatory. If you don't have any room left after having the protein, you can skip the vegetables.

Dieticians categorize meals of this stage into two groups, A and B.

The Diet Groups A & B

Group A: It consists of food items high in their protein content, examples include eggs, low carb high protein yogurt, low fat cottage cheese, egg substitute, tuna (packed in foil/water pouch), salmon (packed in foil/water pouch), Greek-style plain yogurt (they might be sweetened with zero calorie artificial sweeteners), tilapia, ocean perch, flounder, chicken breast (foil pouched, canned or boiled), turkey breast (canned) etc.

Group B: Group B consists of low carb vegetables that you can eat only if you have enough room after consuming 3 ounce of protein. Each meal should not include more than one vegetable and each serving should contain ½ cup of that vegetable. Some of the vegetables you can have in stage 3 are:

- Spinach
- Carrots
- Asparagus
- Green beans
- Beets

- Canned tomatoes
- Mushrooms
- Turnip greens

Sample Menu for Stage 3

Breakfast

- Eggs- 2 (soft boiled, poached or scrambled)
- Low fat cheese- 1 slice
- Mushrooms: ½ cup
- Salt to taste
- Pepper to taste

You can replace 2 eggs with half cup of egg substitute.

Lunch

- Chicken- 3 ounces (boiled, blended)
- Fat free dressing- 2 tablespoons (you can replace it with 1 tablespoon fat free sour cream)
- Green beans or Carrots- ½ cup
- Salt to taste
- Pepper to taste

Dinner

- Salmon or tuna- 3 ounces (packed in water, blended)
- Fat free mayonnaise- 1 tablespoon (you can replace it with ½ tsp spices and herbs)
- Beet or asparagus- ½ cup
- Salt to taste

- Pepper to taste

Stage 4: Low Carb High Protein Diet

After consuming blended food for a couple of weeks, your surgeon will ask you to start following a low carb high protein diet plan. You will have to follow this plan until you lose at least 75% of the excess body weight you are carrying.

Some of the major changes taking place in stage 4 are:

- By this time, your digestive system will be fit enough to tolerate normal consistency foods. So, in this stage, you will be allowed to consume foods of regular consistency.

- Your surgeon will allow you to eat some additional high protein foods, for instance grilled foods. You will get to know about more protein options for stage 4 later in the book.

- Your choices of vegetables will, however, still be limited. You will have to stick to the group B list provided above for a minimum of three months. When in stage 4, you will be allowed to consume fresh cooked and/or frozen vegetables, but will be asked to stay away from raw vegetables (you must do this for the first three months). This is because raw vegetables contain higher percentage of fiber and are thus more difficult to digest. Cut all vegetables you are planning to eat into small pieces and cook them thoroughly to avoid indigestion.

- You should never commit the mistake of eating more than you need. Don't keep eating if you are already full. You can skip or delay a meal if you are not feeling hungry. However, you should try to have at least three meals per day. Maintain a gap of 4 to 6 hours between meals to allow your digestive system to function properly. Don't forget to contact your dietician or surgeon if you are continuously failing to meet your daily protein goals.

- You should never rush when adding new protein sources to your diet. Begin by adding them in very small amounts. If any of those newly introduced foods causes intolerance wait for two weeks before trying it again.

- Don't engage in snacking.

- You should not consume any liquid calorie. Stay away from frozen yogurt, ice cream, fruit juice, smoothies, milk etc.

- Stay away from red meat and pork for at least 6 months. If you fail to lose 75% of the excess body weight you are carrying within 6 months, you should continue to avoid having pork and red meat until you achieve that goal.

- Your diet should not include fruits, potatoes, rice, pasta, breads and bread products (these include tortillas, crackers and cereals) and beans until you get rid of 75% of your excess body weight.

Note: don't start including different additional food items without consulting your surgeon or dietician even after losing 75% of your excess body weight.

Protein Information for Stage 4

- Chew as much as you can (as least 20 times) to allow proper digestion. If you don't chew properly, foods consumed by you will struggle to pass through the tiny stomach opening causing indigestion.

- In this stage 2 you must consume at least 60 grams of protein per day. If you are having three meals a day, each meal should contain 3 ounces (20 grams) of protein. Initially, you can use scales for measuring your foods. However, you will not need them after a few weeks.

- Chicken and turkey breasts can be added to your daily diet (stay away from red meat). You should not have fried or breaded meat.

- You can grill, broil, or bake the lean protein sources mentioned above. However, never have the meat with its skin on (the skin contain high quantity of unhealthy fat).

- Shellfish or fish can be a part of your stage 4 diet. You can opt for crabs, lobsters, shrimps, clams and oysters. One ounce of each of these protein sources contains 35 calories.

- You can have homemade hamburger patties prepared using ground chicken or turkey.

- You can also have salads made using finely chopped and cooked turkey or chicken. Add a tablespoon of fat free mayo or a light salad dressing to make the salad tastier.

- You will get flavored packages of protein sources such as chicken, tuna and salmon in your local store. Read the label of those packages carefully to find out how much carbohydrate the food items contain. If it's' less than 5 g per serving, bring one or two such packages home. This will help you to make your meal more interesting.

After you achieve the target of losing 75% or more of your excess body weight, you should visit your dietician and surgeon for discussing about the food items that you can add to your diet at this point. The basics of your new diet will be same, but a few more calories will be added to it so that you can maintain your body weight successfully. This diet will actually be much more balanced than the diet plans you followed during the previous four stages.

Your dietician might allow you to add pork, veal and beef to your daily meal in limited quantities. This decision will, however, depend on your weight loss goal and percentage. Digesting dark meat is much more difficult than digesting white meat. So, you must chew them properly before swallowing. Ideally, you should chew every bite you take for at least 20 times. Another thing you will have to keep in mind is that you must consume these meats in very small portions as they contain much more (double or may be triple) calories compared to the fish and white meats.

Below are some more tips for making your meals more interesting.

1. You can spice up your proteins in the following ways:

Turkey/chicken: By adding lime/lemon juice, paprika, oregano, sage, rosemary, thyme, tarragon, ginger, marjoram and/or poultry seasoning

Fish: By adding dill, lime/lemon juice, curry powder, dry mustard, pepper, paprika, marjoram and/or cilantro

Beef: By adding thyme, sage, onion, nutmeg, marjoram, garlic and/or bay leaf

Pork: By adding sage, pepper, oregano, onion and/or garlic

2. To spice up vegetables, do the following:

Greens: Add pepper and/or onion

Broccoli: Add rosemary, grated parmesan, lemon juice and/or garlic powder

Cauliflower: Add curry powder, cumin, garlic powder and/or rosemary

Carrots: Add cloves, cinnamon, sage, rosemary, marjoram and/or nutmeg

Green beans: Add oregano, dill, marjoram, lemon juice, thyme, tarragon and/or curry powder

Asparagus: Add garlic powder, parsley, thyme and/or lemon juice

Winter squash: Add onion, nutmeg, ginger and/or cinnamon

Summer squash: Add oregano, curry powder, nutmeg, marjoram, sage, cloves and/or rosemary

Here are a few things you must keep in mind after undergoing gastric bypass surgery:

- To ensure that you are getting all the essential nutrients in right quantities, you must continue taking recommended types and amounts of minerals and vitamins as long as you live after the sleeve gastrectomy. To ensure that the supplements are broken down completely before reaching your digestive system, your surgeon will possibly ask you to consume those essential nutrients in chewable, sugar-free forms. This, in turn, will enable easy digestion and absorption.

- Don't start consuming any additional mineral or vitamin supplement besides the ones mentioned in your prescription without consulting your surgeon or dietician. These professionals are aware of the composition of different nutritional supplements and know which one would be beneficial for you.

- Never take minerals and vitamins in capsule form unless it's a capsule formulated keeping in mind the needs of individuals who have undergone bariatric surgery. You can, however, sprinkle the contents of some mineral and vitamin capsules over your food. This rule applies both for capsules containing powders and gel capsules (instead of sprinkling the gel over food, you can pierce the gel capsules open and swallow the gel).

- Patients who have undergone gastric sleeve surgery are not allowed to consume a whole pill for the rest of their lives. This is because the whole pills can get trapped in their pouch and result in irritation. If these patients continue consuming whole pills, they might even experience ulcer formation.

- Ask your dietician to give you alternatives for every food item you are allowed to eat. This will ensure that your diet doesn't appear monotonous to you.

- It would be a wise decision to use a pill organizer. A pill organizer will not allow you to forget your regular doses of minerals and vitamins. You should prepare a schedule elaborating your monthly, weekly or daily dosages of vitamins.

Chapter 8

Getting Emotionally Adjusted and Motivated

When recovering after sleeve gastrectomy or any other form of bariatric surgery, patients also need to make some emotional adjustments. If you are struggling to adjust to the change emotionally, the following tips will help you.

- You should abide by all recommendations made by your surgeon and dietician meticulously. These include adopting different dietary changes advised by them, taking enough rest, and looking after all your physical needs.

- You should maintain a food diary. Write down what you are eating each day in that diary. This might appear to be a boring job, but will help you immensely in the long run. If you manage to keep track of the foods you are consuming and their effects on your health, you will automatically start feeling more confident and gain more control over your emotions. Your physical health will also improve. This habit will help you understand that you are actually enjoying eating quite a few foods recommended by your dietician.

- Your expectations and goals must be realistic. While for some patients the main goal is getting of medications, others undergo the surgery to get rid of obesity-related physical deformities and disabilities. Whatever you goal or goals may be, jot them down in a diary. Keep modifying them as required.

- It's true that moving on is extremely important, but in this case remembering the past is probably as important. Patients must remember the situation that forced them to take the decision of undergoing the surgery. This will keep them motivated for putting in their best efforts for ensuring that the surgery offers them the desired results.

- Before undergoing the surgery, you must take several pictures of your obese body. Measure all your major body parts such as arms, abdomen, chest, thighs etc. Don't forget to keep some of the clothes (particularly pants) you wear. You should keep taking pictures at regular intervals even after the surgery is done. The pictures will remind you about your success.

  Pre-op garments and measurements are particularly essential during dreaded plateaus. This is the time when we might be losing inches and only pre-op measurements and clothes can help us identify such changes.

- Last, but definitely not the least you should never hesitate to seek help. If you see that you are finding it difficult to adjust to the changes physically and/or emotionally, you should contact your surgeon immediately. You can also seek support from friends, family members, support groups or can undergo psychological counseling. Getting in touch with support groups is particularly beneficial as it helps us to realize that we are not the only people who are facing such issues. This, in turn, provides us with the emotional strength required to fight with different problems related to bariatric surgery. Remember that you have undergone the surgery to improve quality of life and so, you should not shy away from putting in the best efforts.

This Page Has Been Left Blank Intentionally.

Chapter 9

Keys to Successful Weight Loss

There are some dietary habits you must adopt. Please check them out below:

- Stay away from liquid calories.

- Take mineral and vitamin supplements recommended by your dietician and surgeon.

- Keep record of your daily diet.

- Never drink fluids just after eating.

- Don't put more than 6 ounces food on your plate together. If you love seeing a full place in front of your, start using smaller plates instead of the regular-sized plates.

- Begin chewing thoroughly and learn eating slowly.

- You should stop eating before you start feeling too full.

- Your daily fluid intake should be more than 64 ounce. Never gulp liquids. Instead, sip them slowly.

Exercise regularly

A combined workout program of resistance training and aerobic exercises will allow you to lose weight faster and more easily. The combined program will work by increasing your basal metabolic rate or BMR which means you will be losing weight even when sitting idle.

Aerobic exercise: This type of exercise involves brisk physical activities that would require your lungs and heart to work much harder for meeting your body's increased demand for oxygen. Performing aerobic exercises regularly will improve blood circulation and ensure that all your organs receive the nutrients consumed by you. These exercises also help in reducing excess fat stored in your body. Examples of aerobic exercises include jogging, walking, swimming, biking, treadmill. For obese patients, who are trying to lose weight after sleeve gastrectomy, walking, treadmill and swimming are the best options.

Resistance training: Resistance training will increase your muscle mass and make your muscles much stronger. It's unlikely that obese patients will be able to perform free hand strength training exercises. So, for them, the best options would be exercising with free weights, weight machines or resistance bands.

The pointers below show why exercising regularly is important-

• You will be able to achieve your goal weight and then maintain it seamlessly.

• You will experience increase in your endurance and strength.

- Exercise is a mood enhancer.

- It helps in improving skin elasticity.

- Exercise improves mobility and increases flexibility.

- Exercise regularly to experience significant improvement in the functioning of your lungs and heart.

- Exercise promotes sound sleep, increases energy level and lowers blood pressure.

- It improves self-esteem and eliminates anxiety, stress and depression.

- You will be able to quit smoking more easily if you exercise regularly.

- Your life expectancy will also increase.

- You bone and joint health will improve.

- Regular exercise helps in lowering blood sugar levels in diabetics.

When trying to lose weight after the gastric sleeve surgery, you must work out under the supervision of an experienced physical trainer. A workout program should always be started slowly. Increase intensity and time gradually as your body starts getting accustomed to different exercises. Ideally, patients must start exercising prior to the operation and continue with the same workout program post-surgery.

Chapter 10

Tips and Goals for Successful Weight Maintenance

Individuals losing weight through sleeve gastrectomy don't need to undergo regular band fillings like the obese individuals treated with lap band surgery. However, post-surgery and after achieving their weight loss goal, they need to put in significant efforts for maintaining their body weight. For successful weight maintenance after a gastric sleeve surgery, you will have to do the following:

Follow a strict diet plan

You will have to follow new set of dietary guidelines as long as you will live after the surgery. If you again start having all those fried foods and fast foods like you used to do before the operation, you will not be able to keep the weight off.

Exercise regularly

Ideally, you should workout 5 to 6 days per week and each session should last for 30 minutes. If you cannot dedicate so much time for exercising, reduce the number of days. To maintain weight, you will have to exercise at least three times every week. If you are exercising just thrice a week, you should try to keep each session running for a minimum of 45 minutes.

Maintain your mood

It's definitely not possible to be positive all the time. All of us have bad days and people's reactions to such situations tend to vary significantly. Depression often leaves people with a disorder called food addiction. The most common result of the problem is obesity. People with food addiction find solace in food and keep on eating without thinking about their increasing body weight.

If your obesity resulted from food addiction, you must take the necessary step to ensure that you don't fall prey to such disorders again after losing weight through a process like sleeve gastrectomy. You should take notice of your emotional state and mood regularly. Ask yourself whether you are happy and motivated. Find out whether you are abnormally tired. Find out whether you are feeling like spending time with your friends and family members. If answers to these questions reveal that you are again approaching depression, talk to a support group or undergo psychological counseling. Your doctor might help you to get in touch with people and organizations that might help you in this situation.

Wrapping Up!

When an individual undergoes gastric sleeve surgery or sleeve gastrectomy, he needs to follow a series of rules and regulations both before and after the procedure. During this period, these patients are supported by a team of surgeons, mental health experts, nurses, physical trainers, insurance specialists and last, but not least dieticians.

If you want this weight loss surgery to show desired results, you must eat right. Eating right is also important for avoiding postsurgical complications.

Now you know all the basics of the weight loss procedure called gastric sleeve surgery. This procedure can come in handy if you or any of your near or dear ones is fighting obesity.

The success of this surgery depends less on the surgeon, dietician and the hospital and more on the patient. Sleeve gastrectomy fails to show the desired results mostly when patients lose their conviction. So, the most important factor obese individuals should consider before undergoing this procedure is whether they are determined enough to change their lifestyle forever. Weight loss is not the only reward of the surgery. The process also makes patients healthier and more energetic than ever before.

At last, I would like to thank you for reading this book and hope that you will create a new healthier you!

Made in the USA
Middletown, DE
08 July 2016